Early vs. Late Puberty: Effects on Mental and Physical Health

By

Dr. Emily k Pitts

Disclaimer

The material presented in this debate on "Early vs. Late Puberty: Effects on Mental and Physical Health" is meant for general educational purposes only. It is not a replacement for expert medical advice, diagnosis, or treatment. Always seek the assistance of a skilled healthcare provider with any questions you may have regarding a medical condition or before making any decisions relating to your health.

About the Author

Emily K. Pitts is a prominent child psychologist and author with over 15 years of expertise focusing on adolescent development. Her recent book, "Early vs. Late Puberty: Effects on Mental and Physical Health," builds on her considerable clinical experience and research to explore the different implications of pubertal timing. Pitts is known for her approachable writing style and her devotion to helping parents, educators, and healthcare professionals understand and support young people through the problems of puberty. She holds a Ph.D. in developmental psychology and has contributed to various academic journals and conferences on adolescent health.

Table of contents

Conclusion

INTRODUCTION

As a significant developmental stage that denotes the passage from infancy to adulthood, puberty is an important developmental phase. During this time, the human body goes through a number of changes that are biochemical, physical, and emotional in nature. These changes facilitate the process of sexual reproduction. It is possible for the timing of puberty to have a substantial impact on an individual's physical health, psychological well-being, and the social experiences they have. The purpose of this essay is to provide a comprehensive analysis of the meaning of the term "puberty," the distinctions between early and late puberty, and the significance of comprehending the duration of puberty.

Definition of Puberty
After reaching sexual maturity and being capable of reproduction, teenagers go through a

period of time known as puberty. This stage is marked by the stimulation of the hypothalamic-pituitary-gonadal (HPG) axis, leading to the generation of sex hormones such as testosterone in men and estrogen in females. These hormones initiate a cascade of changes, including the development of secondary sexual traits, growth spurts, and variations in body composition.

The onset of puberty is indicated by numerous major milestones. In females, the first symptom is typically thelarche, the growth of breast buds, followed by pubarche, the appearance of pubic hair, and ultimately menarche, the commencement of menstruation. In males, the initial symptom is usually testicular growth, followed by pubarche and the development of other secondary sexual features such as a deeper voice and facial hair.

Explanation of Early and Late Puberty
The time of puberty might vary widely among individuals. While there is a vast range of

normalcy, variations from the usual onset can be characterized as early or late puberty.

Early Puberty (Precocious Puberty)
Early puberty, or precocious puberty, is commonly described as the onset of puberty before the age of 8 in girls and 9 in boys. The causes of early puberty can be multifaceted, including hereditary factors, environmental effects, and specific medical disorders. For instance, exposure to endocrine-disrupting substances, obesity, and some central nervous system illnesses might induce the early beginning of puberty.

The repercussions of early puberty are enormous. Children who experience early puberty generally confront a unique set of obstacles. Physically, they may initially develop taller than their contemporaries, but their growth plates may close early, resulting in a decreased final adult height. Psychologically, early-maturing children may struggle with the emotional and social constraints of seeming older than they are, which can contribute to greater rates of anxiety, sadness, and reduced self-esteem.

Late Puberty (Delayed Puberty)
Delayed puberty is commonly described as the absence of the onset of puberty by age 13 in girls and age 14 in boys. Similar to early puberty, the causes of delayed puberty can be various, ranging from constitutional development delays to more serious underlying medical issues such as hypogonadism, chronic diseases, or starvation.

Children with delayed puberty sometimes suffer tremendous distress owing to their physical immaturity compared to their classmates. This can lead to social isolation, bullying, and a bad self-image. Additionally, the underlying medical issues causing delayed puberty may require specific treatments to address both the delay and the fundamental cause.

Discussion of the Significance of Studying the Timing of Puberty

Understanding the timing of puberty is vital for various reasons, spanning physical health, psychological well-being, and broader societal ramifications.

Physical Health Implications

The timing of puberty has important ramifications for physical health. Early puberty has been associated with many undesirable health outcomes, including an increased risk of metabolic syndrome, type 2 diabetes, cardiovascular disease, and some malignancies. This is partly due to the prolonged period of exposure to sex hormones and the possible relationship with obesity, which is both a cause and a result of early puberty.

Conversely, late puberty can also be associated with health difficulties. Delayed puberty may signal underlying endocrine problems or chronic health concerns that require medical care.

Additionally, those who suffer from delayed puberty might have reduced bone density, leading to an increased risk of osteoporosis and fractures later in life.

Psychological and Social Implications

The psychological influence of the timing of puberty is considerable. Adolescents who mature earlier or later than their classmates sometimes experience substantial social and emotional issues. Early-maturing girls, for instance, are at a higher risk of developing eating disorders, depression, and participating in dangerous behaviors such as substance misuse and early sexual activity. Early-maturing boys could encounter different pressures, such as higher expectations for adult-like behavior, before they are emotionally equipped.

Late-maturing adolescents, on the other hand, often feel low self-esteem and social issues due to their physical immaturity. Boys who mature late may be more vulnerable to bullying and social isolation, while girls may feel self-conscious about their lack of development.

Educational and Societal Implications

The timing of puberty can also have broader educational and societal ramifications. Early-maturing adolescents could struggle academically due to the social and emotional issues they confront, potentially leading to lower educational performance and fewer employment possibilities. Conversely, delayed puberty could hinder school performance due to underlying health difficulties or psychological anguish.

Understanding the timing of puberty and its ramifications can improve public health measures and educational policy. For instance, offering proper sex education and emotional support in schools can help reduce the issues faced by early- or late-maturing teenagers. Additionally, knowledge and early action can enhance health outcomes and boost the well-being of affected people.

In summary, puberty is a key developmental stage with far-reaching ramifications for physical health, psychological well-being, and social results. The timing of puberty, whether early, on-time, or late, has a vital influence in defining these results. By examining the timing of puberty, we can better understand the factors that influence this key phase and develop strategies to support adolescents through these transformations. This understanding is vital for developing healthier, happier, and more resilient individuals capable of handling the challenges of adolescence and beyond.

Chapter 1.

The biological basis of puberty

Puberty marks the transition from childhood to adolescence, a watershed moment marked by rapid physical, hormonal, and psychological transformations. This chapter delves into the complex biological foundations of puberty, focusing on hormonal changes, genetic and environmental influences, and physiological markers that indicate the onset and progression of this developmental stage.

Hormonal Changes

A complex interplay of hormones, which serve as chemical messengers regulating the body's developmental processes, orchestrates the onset of puberty. The main hormones involved in puberty are gonadotropin-releasing hormone (GnRH), luteinizing hormone (LH), follicle-stimulating hormone (FSH), and the sex steroids testosterone and estrogen.

Gonadotropin Releasing Hormone (GnRH): Puberty begins in the hypothalamus, a small brain region responsible for the production of GnRH. GnRH secretion is pulsatile, which means it comes out in bursts rather than a steady stream. This pulsatile release is important because it stimulates the anterior pituitary gland to produce and secrete LH and FSH. Both genetic and environmental cues, such as nutritional status and overall health, influence GnRH secretion.

Luteinizing hormone (LH) and follicle-stimulating hormone (FSH): LH and FSH, also known as gonadotropins, play critical roles in stimulating the gonads—testes in males and ovaries in females. In males, LH causes the Leydig cells in the testes to produce testosterone, the primary male sex hormone. FSH, in conjunction with testosterone, promotes spermatogenesis, or sperm production. In females, FSH promotes the development and maturation of ovarian follicles, each of which contains an egg, whereas LH causes ovulation and the production of estrogen and progesterone.

Sex steroids (testosterone and estrogen): Testosterone and estrogen are responsible for the development of secondary sexual characteristics and reproductive abilities. In males, testosterone promotes the growth of facial and body hair, a deeper voice, and increased muscle mass. Estrogen promotes breast development, hip width, and menstrual cycle regulation in females. Both hormones contribute to the growth spurt and changes in body composition that occur during puberty.

The complex feedback loops between these hormones ensure that puberty occurs in a coordinated manner. For example, rising sex steroid levels eventually inhibit further GnRH, LH, and FSH release, thereby maintaining hormonal balance.

The Impact of Genetics and Environment

A variety of genetic and environmental factors influence the timing and progression of puberty. Understanding these influences helps to explain why pubertal development varies between individuals.

Genetic influences: Genetics plays an important role in determining the onset and progression of puberty. According to studies, the age at which parents reach puberty is frequently associated with their children's pubertal timing. Pubertal timing has been linked to specific genes, such as those that regulate GnRH secretion and the gonads' responsiveness to gonadotropins. Genome-wide association studies (GWAS) have identified numerous genetic loci associated with the age of menarche in girls and voice breaking in boys, demonstrating the polygenic nature of pubertal timing.

Environmental influences: While genetics provides a potential framework for pubertal timing, environmental factors can influence this trajectory. Nutritional status is an important environmental determinant; adequate nutrition is required for energy-intensive processes such as growth and development. Malnutrition or severe caloric restriction can postpone puberty, whereas better nutrition and increased body fat have been linked to earlier pubertal onset.

Endocrine Disruptors: Endocrine disruptors are chemicals in the environment that can interfere with hormonal systems and affect pubertal timing. Certain pesticides, plastics, and industrial chemicals can mimic or block the action of natural hormones, potentially causing puberty to occur earlier or later.

Psychosocial Factors: Stress and psychosocial factors influence pubertal timing. Some studies have linked chronic stress or adverse childhood experiences to an earlier onset of puberty. The exact mechanisms are unknown, but stress hormones such as cortisol may interact with the hormonal pathways that regulate puberty.

Physiological Markers of Puberty

Puberty is characterized by a number of physiological changes that serve as developmental markers. These changes, which frequently occur in a predictable sequence, can be divided into external and internal markers.

External markers include: 1. growth spurt. The adolescent growth spurt, a sudden increase in height and weight, is one of the most obvious signs of puberty. Growth hormone, sex steroids, and insulin-like growth factor-1 (IGF-1) work together to drive this growth spurt. Girls typically experience a growth spurt earlier than boys, often two years before menarche. Boys experience a later growth spurt but gain more height overall.

2. Development of Secondary Sexual Characteristics: These characteristics distinguish males and females but are not directly involved in reproduction.

i. For males: Significant indicators include increased facial and body hair, deepening of the voice, and increased muscle mass. Testicular enlargement is among the first signs of puberty in boys.

ii. In females: Breast development (thelarche) and the start of menstruation (menarche) are important indicators. Hair growth in the pubic and axillary areas occurs, as do changes in body fat distribution.

3. Skin Changes: Androgen-induced increased sebum production causes oily skin and increases the risk of acne. This is a common pubertal change for both genders.

Internal Markers:

1. Reproductive Organ Development: Proper maturation of the reproductive organs is crucial during puberty.

i. In males: Testicular and penile growth, as well as the onset of spermatogenesis, indicate reproductive maturity.

ii. In females: Ovarian maturation, uterine lining development, and the onset of regular menstrual cycles all indicate reproductive capability.

2) Bone Maturation: Puberty causes significant changes to bone structure and density. The growth plates (epiphyses) of long bones gradually close under the influence of sex steroids, signaling the end of the growth spurt and the achievement of adult height.

3. Body Composition Changes: During puberty, the distribution of muscle and fat shifts, influenced by sex steroids. Boys typically gain more muscle mass and have lower body fat than girls, who gain body fat, particularly in the hips, thighs, and breasts.

Puberty is a complex biological process characterized by distinct physiological changes and influenced by genetic and environmental factors. Understanding the biological basis of puberty provides critical information about human development and health. It emphasizes the interaction of our genetic blueprint and environmental influences in shaping the course of growth and maturation. We gain a thorough understanding of puberty by investigating its hormonal, genetic, and environmental dimensions.

Chapter 2
Early Puberty

Definition of the Term and the Age Range That It Encompasses Early puberty, often referred to as precocious puberty, is the onset of the physical and hormonal changes that are associated with puberty occurring at an age that is significantly earlier than the average. Typically, puberty begins between ages 8 and 13 for girls and 9 and 14 for boys. We refer to the onset of puberty as precocious when it occurs before the age of eight in females and before the age of nine in males. Puberty is triggered by the stimulation of the hypothalamic-pituitary-gonadal (HPG) axis, leading to the release of sex hormones that cause the development of secondary sexual traits. These include breast development in girls, testicular enlargement in boys, and the growth of pubic and axillary hair in both sexes.

Additionally, there are considerable growth spurts and changes in body composition during this period.

The Factors That Define the Risk

Several variables contribute to the likelihood of early puberty. These can be generically divided into genetic, environmental, and medicinal factors.

Genetic Factors

Genetics play a vital role in the timing of puberty. Children with a family history of early puberty are more likely to experience it themselves. Genetic abnormalities such as McCune-Albright syndrome and congenital adrenal hyperplasia can potentially promote early puberty.

Environmental Factors: Exposure to some environmental conditions can expedite the beginning of puberty. Endocrine-disrupting chemicals (EDCs) found in pesticides, plastics, and personal care products can imitate or interact with the body's hormone systems, potentially leading to early puberty. Additionally, higher body mass index (BMI) and obesity have been associated with earlier pubertal onset, especially in girls.

Medical Factors

Certain medical disorders and medications might cause early puberty. For example, central nervous system disorders such as tumors or trauma might disrupt the HPG axis. Chronic illnesses and associated treatments, such as those using corticosteroids, may potentially contribute to precocious puberty.

The Effects on One's Physical Health

Early puberty has various ramifications for an individual's physical health, both in the short and long term.

- Short-Term Physical Health Effects The early onset of puberty can lead to rapid skeletal growth and the early closure of growth plates, resulting in a shorter adult stature. Girls may develop menstrual issues, including irregular periods and increased menstrual bleeding, due to the immature hypothalamic-pituitary-ovarian axis. Boys may confront higher hostility and behavioral changes as a result of elevated testosterone levels.

- Long-Term Physical Health Effects Over the long term, early puberty can increase the risk of various health issues. These include polycystic ovarian syndrome (PCOS) in women, which is associated with irregular periods, excessive hair growth, and infertility. Early pubertal onset has also been associated to an increased chance of acquiring type 2 diabetes, cardiovascular disorders, and certain malignancies, such as breast cancer in women and testicular cancer in men.

The Patterns of Growth

The growth patterns of children undergoing early puberty differ dramatically from those of their classmates who endure puberty at a regular age.

Growth Spurts

Children with precocious puberty may undergo an initial growth spurt that leads to an early peak in height velocity. This rapid development phase occurs earlier than in their peers and can result in these children being taller than their classmates initially.

Final Adult Height

Despite the early growth surge, these youngsters generally do not reach their full potential as adults. The early activation of sex hormones accelerates the development of the skeleton and leads to the early closing of growth plates in the bones, which limits further growth in height.

Consequently, children with early puberty may end up shorter than they would have if they had gone through puberty at the regular age.

The Potential for Obesity

Early puberty is associated with an increased risk of obesity. Several mechanisms may contribute to this relationship:

Hormonal Changes

The hormonal changes that occur throughout puberty might impact body composition and fat distribution. Increased levels of estrogen in girls and testosterone in males can lead to changes in fat storage patterns, thereby boosting weight gain and raising the risk of obesity.

Lifestyle Factors

Children who experience early puberty may engage in behaviors that predispose them to weight gain. For instance, kids might adopt adult eating habits earlier than their peers, resulting in increased calorie intake. They may also be more likely to indulge in sedentary activities as they battle with self-esteem issues and social challenges.

Metabolic Changes

Early puberty can produce metabolic changes that raise the probability of developing insulin resistance, a precursor to type 2 diabetes. Insulin resistance can contribute to weight gain and make it more difficult to lose weight, thus increasing the risk of obesity.

The Effects on Long-Term Health Concerns

The long-term health risks connected with early puberty are varied and can impair different elements of an individual's health.

Cardiovascular Health

Early puberty has been linked to an increased risk of cardiovascular illnesses later in life. The hormonal changes throughout puberty can influence lipid profiles, blood pressure, and insulin sensitivity, all of which are risk factors for cardiovascular illnesses.

Bone Health

Although early puberty speeds skeletal growth, it can have severe implications for bone health in the long term. The early closure of growth plates can result in reduced peak bone mass, increasing the risk of osteoporosis and fractures in maturity.

Cancer Risk

Women who have early puberty have an increased risk of acquiring breast cancer. The extended exposure to estrogen is likely to contribute to this elevated risk. Similarly, early puberty in boys has been associated with an increased risk of testicular cancer.

Repercussions on Mental Health

Early puberty can have substantial effects on mental health, altering self-esteem, body image, and the chance of acquiring mental health disorders.

Self-Esteem and Body Image

Children who endure early puberty may feel different from their peers, leading to feelings of isolation and low self-esteem. Girls, in particular, may suffer from body image concerns as they develop secondary sexual features earlier than their classmates. This might result in negative body image and increased self-consciousness.

Risk of Depression and Anxiety

The psychological impact of early puberty can raise the chance of developing sadness and anxiety. Studies have indicated that girls who undergo early puberty are more likely to express symptoms of depression and anxiety than their counterparts who go through puberty at the standard age. Boys, too, can experience greater rates of despair and anxiety, but this is less well documented.

Social Challenges : The social barriers faced by children undergoing early puberty can be severe and can further exacerbate the mental health issues they may suffer.

Peer Relationships

Children with early puberty may find it tough to relate to their peers, who may still be in the prepubescent stage. This might lead to social isolation and trouble building friendships. Girls may encounter mocking or bullying owing to their early physical development, while boys may feel pressure to conform to masculine stereotypes associated with higher testosterone levels.

Academic Performance

The social and emotional issues associated with early puberty can significantly influence academic achievement. Children who are battling with self-esteem, body image difficulties, and mental health concerns may find it difficult to concentrate on their studies, leading to a reduction in academic performance.

Risky Behaviors

Early puberty has been related to an increased possibility of engaging in dangerous behaviors, such as substance use, early sexual activity, and delinquency. The combination of hormonal changes, psychological stress, and societal influences can contribute to this higher risk.

Early puberty is a complex disorder with wide-ranging impacts on an individual's physical and mental health, as well as their social well-being. Understanding the variables that contribute to early puberty, the patterns of growth, and the possible long-term health consequences is vital for providing appropriate support and therapies for affected children. Healthcare practitioners, parents, and educators must work together to address the particular issues experienced by children experiencing early puberty. By establishing a supportive environment and promoting healthy habits, it is possible to offset some of the negative effects associated with early pubertal onset and help

these children thrive despite the problems they
may confront.

Chapter 3

Late Puberty

Definition and Age Distribution

When puberty occurs later than the usual range of ages, late puberty, often referred to as delayed puberty, is the absence of the physical and chemical changes associated with puberty. Between the ages of 8 and 13 for females and 9 and 14 for boys, puberty often sets in. Delay in puberty is the state in which these changes have not begun by the age of 14 for boys and 13 for girls. The absence of secondary sexual features, such as breast growth in girls and testicular enlargement in boys, within the anticipated timeframe is the defining feature of delayed puberty. The physical and mental health of an individual may suffer greatly as a result of this delay.

The Elements That Determine the Danger

Genetic, environmental, and medical factors are among the many variables that can increase the likelihood of late puberty.

Genetic Elements

In terms of when puberty occurs, genetics is a major factor. Children who have a family history of delayed puberty are likely to follow a similar trend. Delayed puberty can also result from genetic abnormalities like Turner syndrome in girls and Klinefelter syndrome in boys. Further causes of late pubertal onset include mutations in genes related to the control of the hypothalamic-pituitary-gonadal (HPG) axis.

Environmental Aspects

There is a big impact that environmental factors have on when puberty occurs. Chronic sickness and malnutrition are major causes of delayed puberty. Malnourishment and insufficient calorie intake, frequently observed in eating disorders like anorexia nervosa, can prevent proper pubertal development.

Excessive physical exercise can also postpone puberty, particularly in sports that prioritize low body weight.

Health Concerns

A number of illnesses can cause a delay in puberty. Chronic conditions that affect normal growth and development, such as renal illness, inflammatory bowel disease, and cystic fibrosis, might postpone puberty. In addition to causing disruptions to normal puberty timing, endocrine diseases include growth hormone insufficiency and hypothyroidism. Furthermore, some drugs can prevent pubertal growth, such as glucocorticoids prescribed for long-term conditions.

The Impact on Physical Well-Being

There are several effects of delayed puberty on a person's physical health, influencing both short- and long-term results.

Direct Impact on Physical Health

Compared to their classmates, children who suffer from delayed puberty typically grow at slower rates. This may result in reduced stature and a delayed gain of strength and muscle mass. Boys may not have the pubertal development hallmarks of voice deepening and body and facial hair growth, and girls may not experience menstruation until much later in life.

Long-Term Impacts on Physical Health

Physical health may suffer long-term consequences from delayed puberty. The effect on bone health, which raises the risk of osteoporosis later in life, is one major worry. The absence of sex hormones at crucial stages of bone formation can lead to a decrease in peak bone mass, making people more vulnerable to fractures and problems with bone density.

The Growth Patterns Compared to their counterparts who reach puberty within the usual age range, children who experience delayed puberty exhibit very different growth patterns.

Reduced Rates of Growth

The growth rates of children who experience delayed puberty are often slower than those of their contemporaries. They frequently lag behind in height and weight, giving the impression that they are smaller and less physically mature.

Recovering Growth

Children who have delayed puberty frequently go through a period of catch-up growth once puberty eventually commences. The body tries to reach its genetic potential for stature, which is characterized by a sudden increase in height. But not everyone catches up to their classmates in terms of height, and there might be differences in the amount of catch-up growth.

Osteoporosis Risk

The increased risk of osteoporosis is one of the most important long-term health issues linked to delayed puberty. Weakened bones and a higher risk of fractures are the hallmarks of osteoporosis. Sex hormones are important for both the production and preservation of bones, and they have a significant impact on the growth of bone mass.

Postponed Bone Formation

The spike in sex hormones that occurs throughout puberty—specifically, testosterone in boys and estrogen in girls—enhances bone density and encourages bone growth. Lack of these hormones throughout crucial stages of bone growth in delayed puberty might cause decreased peak bone mass and delayed maturity of the bones.

Effect on Bone Health

Over Time Since delayed puberty results in a lower peak bone mass during the formative years, individuals with delayed puberty are more likely to develop osteoporosis later in life. As individuals get older, this may make them more vulnerable to fractures and problems with their bone density.

Long-Term Medical Results

Delayed puberty has long-term health consequences that go beyond bone health and can affect a person's general wellbeing in a number of ways.

Heart and Circulatory Systems

There is evidence linking postponed puberty to a higher lifetime risk of cardiovascular illnesses. Delay in puberty can cause hormonal abnormalities that impact blood pressure, glucose metabolism, and lipid profiles—all of which are cardiovascular disease risk factors.

Health of the Reproductive System

Delays in puberty might cause irregular menstruation and problems with fertility in later life for girls. Inadequate maturation of the reproductive system may result in difficulties getting pregnant and keeping a pregnancy. Boys who suffer delayed puberty may have fewer sperm and be less fertile.

Health Metabolic

Postponed puberty may have an impact on metabolic health, raising the possibility of type 2 diabetes and metabolic syndrome. Insulin resistance and poor glucose metabolism might result from the hormonal changes brought on by delayed puberty.

Effects on Mental Well-Being

Postponing puberty can have significant negative effects on mental health, including altered body image, low self-esteem, and an increased chance of mental health problems.

Body Image and Self-Esteem

Children who have delayed puberty frequently have problems with their bodies and their self-esteem. In comparison to their peers, they could feel self-conscious about their lower stature and lack of physical development. Low self-worth and feelings of inadequacy may result from this.

Anxiety and Depression

Risk Delay in puberty can have a psychological consequence that raises the likelihood of developing anxiety and despair. Research indicates that children who undergo delayed puberty are more likely than their classmates who go through puberty within the standard age range to express symptoms of anxiety and despair.

Social Difficulties

Children who experience delayed puberty may suffer significant social hurdles, which can worsen whatever mental health problems they may already be facing.

Interactions with Peers

Children who experience delayed puberty may find it difficult to relate to their peers since they are going through the emotional and physical changes that come with puberty. Social isolation and trouble making friends may result from this. Because of their slow   physical development, they could also be the victim of bullying or teasing.

Academic Achievement

A delayed puberty can cause social and emotional difficulties that can affect a person's academic achievement. Children who experience difficulties with their self-worth, body image, or mental health may find it challenging to focus on their academics, which can result in a drop in their academic performance.

Dangerous Actions

An increased chance of participating in dangerous behaviors, such as substance abuse and delinquency, has been associated with delayed puberty. This elevated risk may result from a confluence of hormonal fluctuations, psychological stress, and societal influences.

Final Thoughts The complicated issue of delayed puberty can have a variety of implications for a person's social, emotional, and physical well-being. It is essential to comprehend the growth patterns, the circumstances that lead to delayed puberty, and the possible long-term health issues in order to provide the affected children with the right assistance and solutions. Collaboratively, schools, parents, and healthcare professionals can better meet the special needs of children who are experiencing delayed puberty. It is feasible to lessen some of the negative impacts of delayed pubertal onset and support these kids in thriving despite any obstacles they may face by creating a friendly atmosphere and encouraging healthy activities. It is crucial to guarantee the timely detection and assistance of children experiencing delayed puberty. A good management strategy for the illness can involve regular growth and development monitoring in conjunction with the right kind of medical and psychological assistance. Delay in puberty can also reduce some of the stress and anxiety that accompany it by offering information and assistance to the afflicted youngsters and their families. To sum up, delayed puberty is a complex disorder that has repercussions for social, emotional, and physical health. We can enhance the long-term health results and general well-being of those who experience delayed puberty by comprehending and addressing the different elements that contribute to this condition. With an all-encompassing strategy that incorporates social, psychological, and medical support, we can successfully guide children who experience delayed puberty through their development and help them enjoy happy, satisfying lives.

Chapter 4

Comparative Analysis

An Introduction to the Topic Puberty is a vital developmental stage characterized by considerable physical, emotional, and psychological changes. While the date of puberty can vary greatly among individuals, early and late puberty both bring unique challenges and effects. This chapter gives a comparative review of early and late puberty, focusing on parallels in mental health outcomes, differences in physical health outcomes, and gender variations in the impacts of puberty timing.

Similarities in Mental Health Outcomes

Both early and late puberty can severely impair mental health. Despite the varied timeframes, people experiencing either can share common psychological issues and effects.

Self-Esteem and Body Image

Children facing either early or late puberty may deal with self-esteem and body image concerns. Those who mature sooner than their contemporaries may feel out of place due to their rapid physical development, leading to feelings of humiliation or self-consciousness. Conversely, children with delayed puberty may feel inadequate or frightened about their lack of physical growth compared to their classmates. Both populations can have a negative body image, hurting their general self-esteem.

Risk of Depression and Anxiety

The psychological stress associated with being out of sync with peers can lead to increased risks of depression and anxiety for both early and late development. Early-maturing youngsters may suffer social pressures and bullying, contributing to feelings of isolation and anxiety. Similarly, late-maturing youngsters may endure social rejection and teasing, which can contribute to melancholy and heightened anxiety levels.

Research indicates that both early and late puberty might disturb normal psychological development, increasing susceptibility to mood disorders.

Social Challenges

Social problems are frequent for youngsters experiencing either early or late puberty. Early learners may struggle with building relationships with peers who are at various developmental levels, resulting in feelings of alienation. They could also be subject to unreasonable expectations and duties due to their more mature appearance. Late developers, on the other hand, may be stigmatized or excluded from peer groups, affecting their capacity to create connections and social networks. These social challenges can contribute to long-term issues with social anxiety and relationship-building.

Differences in Physical Health Outcomes

While there are commonalities in the psychological implications of early and late puberty, the physical health outcomes can differ dramatically between the two groups. Early Puberty

Growth Patterns Children experiencing early puberty often have a rapid initial growth spurt. However, the early activation of sex hormones can lead to an early closure of growth plates in the bones, resulting in a shorter adult stature than their contemporaries, who mature at a regular age.

Obesity

Early puberty is associated with an increased risk of obesity. The hormonal changes during early puberty can lead to changes in body composition and fat distribution, increasing the probability of weight gain. Additionally, children who mature early may adopt adult eating habits and sedentary lifestyles earlier, contributing to an increased risk of obesity.

Long-Term Health Concerns

Early puberty has been linked to various long-term health risks, including cardiovascular illnesses, type 2 diabetes, and some cancers such as breast and testicular cancer. The extended exposure to sex hormones is likely to contribute to these higher risks.

Late puberty

Growth Patterns Children with delayed puberty often have slower growth rates compared to their peers. However, as puberty begins, adolescents often endure a period of catch-up growth, resulting in a substantial increase in height. Despite this catch-up growth, individuals may not achieve the same height as their classmates who mature at the regular age.

Bone Health

One of the most serious long-term health issues connected with delayed puberty is an increased risk of osteoporosis. The delayed exposure to sex hormones throughout important times of bone growth can result in decreased peak bone mass, increasing vulnerability to fractures and bone density difficulties later in life.

Reproductive Health

Delayed puberty might result in reproductive health complications. For girls, this may involve menstrual irregularities and reproductive issues. Boys may experience diminished sperm production and lower fertility. The delayed development of the reproductive system can have permanent implications for an individual's capacity to conceive and maintain pregnancies.

Gender Differences in Puberty Timing Effects

The timing of puberty can have varied implications for boys and girls, reflecting the gender-specific nature of hormonal changes and societal expectations.

Early Puberty

Girls

Girls who experience early puberty are more likely to confront substantial psychological and social issues. Early-maturing females frequently experience heightened risks of depression, anxiety, and low self-esteem due to their advanced physical development and the consequent societal expectations. They may also be susceptible to sexual harassment and exploitation, leading to significant psychological suffering. Physically, early puberty in girls is connected with higher risks of obesity, type 2 diabetes, cardiovascular illnesses, and breast cancer. The early commencement of menstruation can also contribute to monthly irregularities and polycystic ovarian syndrome (PCOS), compromising long-term reproductive health.

Boys

Early-maturing boys may first appear to profit from their accelerated development, often being seen as more handsome and competent by peers and adults. However, these perceived advantages also come with increased pressure and expectations to conform to adult-like habits. This can lead to behavioral difficulties, including increased hostility and risk-taking behaviors. Physically, guys who experience early puberty may also suffer from health hazards such as obesity and testicular cancer. The early growth spurt can result in a lower adult stature due to the premature closing of growth plates.

Late puberty

Girls

Girls who have delayed puberty may battle with feelings of inadequacy and low self-esteem due to their lack of physical development compared to their peers. They may endure social rejection and taunting, causing heightened anxiety and sadness. Physically, late puberty in girls might result in reduced peak bone mass, increasing the risk of osteoporosis. Reproductive health difficulties, such as menstrual abnormalities and fertility problems, are also common. The delayed onset of menstruation can lead to long-term issues with reproductive health.

Boys

Boys who undergo delayed puberty often confront substantial social and psychological issues. A lack of physical development can contribute to feelings of humiliation and low self-esteem. They may be susceptible to teasing and bullying, adding to the increased risks of sadness and anxiety. Physically, boys with delayed puberty may endure decreased development rates but often undergo catch-up growth once puberty begins. However, they may still be shorter than their contemporaries. Delayed puberty can also damage bone health, increasing the risk of osteoporosis. Additionally, reproductive health concerns, such as diminished sperm production and poorer fertility, might emerge from delayed development of the reproductive system.

The timing of puberty, whether early or late, brings distinct challenges and outcomes that can greatly impact an individual's physical, mental, and social well-being. While both early and late puberty share parallels in mental health consequences, such as increased chances of sadness, anxiety, and low self-esteem, the physical health effects might differ dramatically. Early puberty is connected with a rapid first growth spurt, a higher risk of obesity, and long-term health risks such as cardiovascular illnesses and some malignancies. Late puberty, on the other hand, is connected to slower growth rates, a higher risk of osteoporosis, and reproductive health difficulties. Gender differences in the consequences of puberty timing further confuse the situation. Girls who experience early puberty suffer heightened risks of psychological discomfort, obesity, and reproductive health difficulties, while boys may encounter increased social demands and behavioral issues. Conversely, girls with delayed puberty struggle with feelings of inadequacy and greater risks of osteoporosis, while boys endure substantial social and psychological obstacles and may have reproductive health issues. Understanding these complications is vital for offering appropriate support and interventions for those experiencing early or late puberty. By establishing a supportive environment and promoting healthy habits, it is possible to offset some of the negative impacts associated with abnormal pubertal timing and help individuals navigate this key developmental stage effectively.

Chapter 5

Longitudinal Studies and Research Findings

puberty is characterized by changes in the body, mind, and social interactions. Comprehending its complexities necessitates extensive investigation, sometimes carried out via longitudinal research. These long-term follow-up studies provide valuable information about the start, development, and aftermath of puberty. This chapter explores important longitudinal studies, including their approaches, results, drawbacks, and potential avenues for further investigation.

Key studies and their findings

1. The Parents and Children Avon Longitudinal Study (ALSPAC) One well-known longitudinal study with roots in the UK is the Avon

Longitudinal Study of Parents and Children (ALSPAC), popularly referred to as the Children of the Nineties study. Established in 1991, ALSPAC monitors the growth and well-being of infants born in the Avon region, offering an abundance of information on several facets of adolescence

Results:

i. Age at Puberty: Understanding the erratic nature of puberty and its timing has greatly benefited ALSPAC. It has determined the elements that impact puberty onset, including genetic impacts, environmental exposures, and fetal growth.

ii. Psychology: According to the study, early puberty is associated with a higher chance of mental health problems, such as anxiety and sadness, especially in girls.

iii. Wellness of Body:The results of ALSPAC emphasize the link between early puberty and increased chances of obesity and cardiovascular problems in later life.

2. The Adolescent to Adult Health National Longitudinal Study (Add Health) A large-scale U.S. study called the National Longitudinal Study of Adolescent to Adult Health (Add Health) got underway in the middle of the 1990s. It focuses on the social, behavioral, and health outcomes of a nationally representative sample of adolescents as they transition into adulthood.

Results:

i. Socioeconomic Factors: In addition, research has shown that socioeconomic level (SES) influences the beginning and course of puberty, with lower SES being associated with earlier pubertal development.

ii. At-Risk Actions: According to the study, adolescents who are still developing have a higher propensity to participate in harmful activities, including substance abuse and early sexual engagement.

iii. Health Trajectories: Add Research suggests that a higher risk of adult metabolic syndrome and cardiovascular diseases is associated with early puberty.

3. Heart Study of Bogalusa Initiated in 1973, the Bogalusa Heart Study is a groundbreaking investigation that looks at cardiovascular risk factors from childhood to maturity. This Bogalusa, Louisiana, study has shed light on the relationship between childhood health and adult cardiovascular health.

Results:

i. Obesity and Puberty: The Bogalusa Heart Study has shown a high correlation, particularly in females, between childhood obesity and the early beginning of puberty.

ii. Health in the Long Run: Research indicates that obesity in childhood and early puberty greatly raises the risk of cardiovascular disease and type 2 diabetes in later life.

4. The Ireland Study of Growing Up A national longitudinal study, Growing Up in Ireland, tracks two cohorts of Irish children, one from infancy to childhood and the other from childhood to adolescence.

Results:

i. Influences from Family and Environment: The study places a strong emphasis on how environmental factors and family dynamics affect the onset and course of puberty.

ii. Academic Results: There is evidence linking early puberty to worse academic outcomes and increased rates of school absences, especially in females.

Methodologies used in Research

Employed To guarantee solid and trustworthy results, longitudinal research on puberty uses a variety of approaches. Important techniques consist of:

1. Cohort Research Cohort studies monitor a population of people over time who have a common attribute, such as age or geography. With this method, researchers may see how different factors affect the beginning and course of puberty.

Advantages: Cohort studies offer comprehensive, continuous data that can pinpoint long-term consequences and causal links. Difficulties: They need a lot of resources, including money, time, and participant retention initiatives.

2. Using Mixed Methods Mixed-methods approaches, which combine quantitative and qualitative data collection techniques, provide a thorough understanding of puberty. Hormone levels and physical measures are examples of quantitative data; questionnaires and interviews

are examples of qualitative data. Strengths: This method captures both quantifiable changes and individual experiences, offering a comprehensive picture of puberty.

Difficulties:

It can be difficult and time-consuming to integrate and analyze different types of data.

3. Studies that Cross-Section Cross-sectional studies are not strictly longitudinal, but they do supplement longitudinal research by offering glimpses of many age groups at one particular moment in time. These studies aid in identifying patterns and distinctions connected to age.

Advantages: Compared to longitudinal investigations, cross-sectional studies are speedier and less expensive. Difficulties: They are unable to monitor individual developmental trajectories or prove causation.

4. Measurements of Biological and Biometric Data In addition to biological samples to test hormone levels and genetic markers, longitudinal studies on puberty often include biometric data, such as height, weight, and body mass index (BMI).

Advantages: These impartial assessments offer precise and measurable information on physical growth.

Difficulties: Biological sample collection and storage can be expensive and logistically difficult.

Limitations and Future Research Directions

Longitudinal studies on puberty have various limitations and obstacles despite their strengths, which need to be addressed to improve future research.

1. Retention of Participants Sustaining participant engagement over prolonged periods

of time presents considerable difficulty. Results from attrition may be skewed if some groups are more likely to discontinue. Remedy: To increase retention rates, researchers might employ tactics including consistent follow-ups, rewards, and preserving solid participant-researcher connections.

2. Intensity of Resources Financial, logistical, and human resources are major requirements for longitudinal investigations. Getting steady support over a long period of time is frequently challenging.

Remedy: One way to lessen the impact of resource limitations is through cooperative initiatives, multi-site investigations, and integration with current data sources.

3. Ethical Points to Take Research involving minors and young adults must handle a number of difficult ethical issues, such as informed consent, privacy, and the study's possible psychological effects.

Solution:

Participants' needs for support services, continuous consent, and adherence to strict ethical criteria can all help to allay these worries.

4. Improvements in Methodology and Technology The swift progress of technology and research approaches brings with them both advantages and disadvantages. While it might be challenging, staying current with new instruments and methods is necessary for reliable research.

Solution: Ongoing instruction and cooperation with technological specialists can guarantee that researchers efficiently take advantage of the most recent developments.

5. Generalizability and Diversity The lack of diversity in the participant populations of many longitudinal studies can have an impact on how broadly applicable the results are. Remedy:

It is possible to increase the applicability of research findings across many groups by designing studies with representative and diverse samples and by performing cross-cultural research.

6. Including Additional Variables New insights on puberty are available from emerging study domains, including microbiomics and epigenetics. It can be difficult, though, to incorporate these variables into already-completed research.

Remedy: Flexible study designs and interdisciplinary collaboration allow for the addition of new variables without interfering with present research.

Final Thoughts Studies with a longitudinal design offer significant insights into the intricate process of puberty. The Bogalusa Heart Study, ALSPAC, Add Health, Growing Up in Ireland, and other important research have enhanced our understanding of the onset, course, and long-term effects of puberty on health and well-being. These researchers' methods, which range from mixed-methods approaches to cohort studies, provide thorough and trustworthy data. But researchers also have to deal with issues including participant retention, resource limitations, moral dilemmas, diversity requirements, and technology integration. Subsequent investigations ought to concentrate on resolving these constraints and investigating novel paths, such as the influence of contemporary environmental elements, the function of genetics and epigenetics, and the impact of digital and social media on puberty. We can improve future generations' health outcomes and get a deeper understanding of puberty by expanding the research scope and refining the methodology.

Chapter 6

Interventions and Support

puberty is characterized by profound changes in one's physical, emotional, and psychological makeup. Children go through this period of transition from childhood to adolescence, encountering a variety of difficulties that call for extensive support networks. This chapter examines a range of medical therapies, psychological therapy, and support systems for controlling puberty, in addition to the critical responsibilities that families and schools play.

Medical Interventions

When it comes to early or delayed puberty and related health problems, medical interventions are crucial for regulating some parts of the process. By treating any difficulties that may occur, these therapies seek to ensure that children proceed through puberty at a healthy and acceptable pace.

1. Hormone treatment One popular medical strategy for managing puberty is hormone therapy. There are several ways to use it, based on what each person needs.

a. Postponing Early Puberty: Hormone therapy can postpone further growth until a more suitable age in situations of premature puberty, which is defined as puberty starting before the ages of 8 for girls and 9 for boys. Usually, this entails using analogs of gonadotropin-releasing hormone (GnRH), which inhibit the production of hormones that cause puberty.

Features: Postponing puberty can mitigate psychological effects, lower the likelihood of short adult stature, and harmonize physical growth with social and emotional development.

Dangers and Things to Think About:

Modest mood swings, headaches, and possible effects on bone density are all possible adverse effects. It is essential to have regular medical monitoring.

b. Stemming Off the Puberty: Hormone therapy can promote the development of secondary sexual traits in those who are suffering from delayed puberty, which is defined as not showing any indications of puberty by the age of 13 for girls and 14 for boys. Usually, this entails giving out testosterone or estrogen.

Features: Puberty induction can support healthy growth patterns, lessen psychological stress, and assist physical development by matching peers.

Dangers and Things to Think About:

Acne, mood fluctuations, and increases in cholesterol levels are possible side effects. Monitoring over an extended period of time is required to guarantee proper dosage and reduce hazards.

2. Handling Medical Conditions Puberty may be impacted by some medical problems, such as congenital adrenal hyperplasia (CAH) or polycystic ovarian syndrome (PCOS). Symptom management and hormone modulation are common medical therapies for these diseases.

a. PCOS, or polycystic ovarian syndrome: Acne, excessive hair growth, and irregular menstrual cycles can all be symptoms of PCOS. Treatments for acne and hair development frequently involve anti-androgen drugs and oral contraceptives to control menstruation. Benefits include decreased hirsutism and acne, regularized menstruation, and maybe avoiding long-term consequences, including diabetes.

Dangers and Things to Think About: Changes in mood, nausea, and weight gain are possible side effects. Follow-up appointments with doctors are crucial.

b. Hyperplasia Adrenal (CAH) at Birth: The hereditary condition known as CAH affects the adrenal glands' ability to produce hormones.

Usually used as a form of treatment, corticosteroids replenish lost hormones and treat symptoms. Reduced danger of adrenal crises, enhanced growth and development, and normalized hormone levels are some of the benefits. Dangers and Things to Think About: Side effects from long-term corticosteroid treatment include weight gain, hypertension, and weakening of the bones. It is necessary to monitor continuously.

Psychological Support and Counseling

Due to the profound emotional and psychological changes that accompany puberty, teenagers need psychological support and therapy to get through this difficult time.

1. Private Counseling

Teenagers who seek individual counseling can safely share their emotions, worries, and fears related to puberty. It aids in their comprehension of the changes they are going through and the creation of coping mechanisms.

Benefits include: higher self-esteem, decreased anxiety and sadness, improved coping mechanisms, and improved emotional control.

Method: Counselors address specific concerns and promote resilience through a variety of therapeutic strategies, including cognitive-behavioral therapy (CBT).

2. Group counseling Adolescents can talk about their experiences with peers who are going through comparable transitions in group therapy. It normalizes puberty and strengthens ties to the community. Benefits include shared coping mechanisms, enhanced social skills, fewer feelings of loneliness, and peer support.

Method: Common puberty-related subjects, including body image, peer pressure, and identity formation, are frequently the focus of group sessions.

3. Family Guidance Working with the entire family to address puberty-related concerns is the goal of family therapy. It facilitates better

communication, conflict resolution, and the development of a loving home. Strengthened ties within the family, more empathy and understanding, and strengthened support networks are the benefits.

Approach: To investigate dynamics and promote constructive changes, therapists employ strategies like family systems therapy.

4. Counseling in Schools When it comes to providing psychological support, schools are essential. School counselors can provide workshops on subjects relevant to puberty in addition to individual and group sessions.

Advantages: Quick access to assistance, less stigma, and alignment with learning objectives.

Approach: School-based initiatives frequently incorporate instruction on stress reduction, emotional control, and fostering positive connections.

Role of Family and School

It is impossible to overestimate the importance of families and schools in helping teenagers through puberty. In order to provide the required emotional, psychological, and educational support, both environments are essential.

1. The Function of the Family Adolescents receive much of their support from their families. They are responsible for encouraging healthy behaviors, facilitating open communication, and offering emotional support.

a. Help with Emotions: Families can provide teenagers with the compassion, empathy, and reassurance they need to help them through the emotional upheaval of puberty. Important elements are to validate their sentiments and to actively listen to them.

Advantages: Less stress and anxiety, more self-esteem, and a more solid sense of stability. Strategies: Provide correct information, encourage candid discussion about issues associated with puberty, and provide an example of healthy coping mechanisms.

b. Encouraging Honest Talk: It's critical to provide a space where teenagers feel at ease talking about their experiences. Clear and honest communication helps dispel myths and delivers reliable facts. Stronger parent-child connections, less stigma and shame, and better-informed teenagers are the benefits.

Tips: Talk to children about puberty, speak to them in a language that suits their age, and be available to answer any queries or concerns they may have.

c. Encouraging Well-Being Actions: Families can help shape the health habits of teenagers by encouraging a healthy diet, frequent exercise, and enough sleep. Making healthy lifestyle choices can help lessen the psychological and physical effects of puberty.

Advantages: Better mental and physical health, less risk of obesity and related disorders, and enhanced emotional stability.

Tips: Set an example of good health, include teenagers in meal preparation and exercise, and create schedules that give sleep and self-care a priority.

2. The Function of Education For teenagers to receive an education, psychological support, and a supportive social environment, schools are essential. They are responsible for creating a supportive school climate, providing counseling services, and putting comprehensive health education programs into action. Programs for Health Education:

a. In-depth health education programs address puberty's social, emotional, and physical elements. They debunk myths and misconceptions while offering correct facts. Benefits include: educated and ready teens; less confusion and worry; and encouragement of healthy habits.

Strategies: Include parents in the educational process, incorporate interactive and interesting teaching techniques, and incorporate puberty education into the curriculum.

b. Services for Counseling: When it comes to offering psychological support, school counselors are essential. They provide crisis intervention, group and individual counseling, and referral services. Benefits include early problem detection, easily accessible support, and the advancement of mental health and wellbeing. Strategies: Establish appropriate counselor-to-student ratios, offer education on topics linked to puberty, and foster a private, encouraging atmosphere.

c. A Culture of Support at School: A healthy school climate promotes a feeling of security and belonging, both of which are essential during adolescence. Schools can put into place procedures and policies that support respect and inclusivity.

Advantages: Less harassment and bullying, better mental health, and higher academic achievement. Strategies: Encourage peer support groups, support anti-bullying initiatives, and involve kids in fostering a positive school climate.

Final Thoughts Puberty is a complicated and demanding time that calls for a variety of support networks. Adolescents can effectively navigate this stage with the assistance of medical therapies, psychological support and counseling, and the roles that families and schools play. Puberty proceeds in a healthy and acceptable manner, thanks to medical interventions like hormone therapy and condition management. Adolescents can better manage the emotional and psychological shifts they go through with the help of psychological therapy and counseling. Families and schools provide the fundamental support networks that encourage healthy growth and wellbeing in the interim. By combining these strategies, we can build an all-encompassing support system that caters to the various needs of teenagers going through puberty, ultimately helping to develop a generation that is healthier, more resilient, and better adjusted.

Chapter 7

Case Studies

Puberty is a vital era of human development characterized by a range of physical, emotional, and psychological changes. The time of puberty can vary substantially among individuals, with some experiencing early or late onset. This chapter includes thorough case studies of early and late puberty, assessing their ramifications and the lessons learned.

Examples of Early Puberty

Early puberty, also known as precocious puberty, occurs when the signs of puberty develop earlier than the average age range. The following case studies demonstrate the experiences and challenges faced by individuals with early puberty.

Case Study 1: Emily Background:

Emily was an eight-year-old girl living in a suburban environment. She was the eldest of three siblings, and her family had no documented history of early puberty. Emily was an active and sociable child, excelling in both school and sports.

Onset of Puberty:Emily's parents detected signs of puberty when she was barely seven years old. She began developing breast buds and experiencing a rapid increase in height. Her pediatrician confirmed the early beginning of puberty through physical examination and hormone tests.

Challenges: Physical Discomfort: Emily endured physical discomfort due to the rapid growth of her breasts and the commencement of menstrual cycles by the age of eight.

Psychological Impact: The early physical changes created severe psychological suffering. Emily felt self-conscious and separated from her peers, who had not yet reached puberty.

Social Difficulties: Emily faced ridicule and bullying at school because of her rapid physical development. This led to a deterioration in her academic performance and social participation.

Interventions: Emily's pediatrician directed her to a pediatric endocrinologist, who prescribed GnRH analogs to postpone further pubertal growth. She also underwent psychological counseling to help her cope with her emotional and social problems.

Outcomes:

Medical: The hormone medication effectively postponed future development, allowing Emily to grow at a more usual pace.

Psychological: Counseling helped Emily establish coping strategies and increase her self-esteem. She also received help from her school, which established anti-bullying measures.

Case Study 2: John Background: John was a nine-year-old boy from an urban environment. He was an only kid and had a family history of early puberty, with his father having similar trends during childhood.

Onset of Puberty: John began showing signs of puberty at the age of eight, including testicular enlargement and the growth of pubic hair. His fast bodily alterations were confirmed by an endocrinologist.

Challenges: Physical Changes: John underwent fast growth, culminating in an early growth spurt. However, this also led to the early closure of his growth plates, impacting his final adult height.

Emotional Stress: The early beginning of puberty produced emotional stress. John struggled with mood swings and heightened anxiety.

Behavioral Issues: John demonstrated increasing anger and trouble concentrating, influencing his behavior at home and school.

Interventions: John was prescribed GnRH analogs to slow down the progression of puberty. He also attended counseling sessions to address his mental and behavioral concerns.

Outcomes:Medical: The intervention successfully postponed future pubertal development, allowing John to reach a more typical growth trajectory.

Emotional and Behavioral: Counseling helped John regulate his emotions and improve his behavior. His parents and teachers were active in providing a supportive environment.

Examples of Late Puberty

Late puberty, or delayed puberty, happens when the indications of puberty are not present in the traditional age range. The following case studies reflect the experiences of people with late puberty and the associated issues.

Case Study 3: Sarah

Background: Sarah was a fifteen-year-old girl from a rural location. She was the youngest of four siblings, all of whom had experienced typical puberty. Sarah was an intellectually oriented student but struggled with self-esteem issues relating to her physical development. Onset of Puberty: Sarah had not developed any secondary sexual features by the age of fourteen. Her pediatrician conducted a complete evaluation and diagnosed her with constitutional delay of growth and puberty (CDGP). Challenges:

Physical Development: Sarah was much shorter and less developed than her contemporaries, leading to feelings of inadequacy.

Psychological Impact: The delay in puberty produced severe psychological anguish. Sarah felt self-conscious and nervous about her physical appearance. Social Isolation: Sarah's delayed growth led to social isolation, as she felt out of place among her peers. Interventions: Sarah's physician prescribed a brief course of low-dose estrogen to stimulate pubertal development. She also underwent psychiatric counseling to address her self-esteem and anxiety difficulties.

Outcomes: Medical: The hormone therapy successfully triggered pubertal growth, and Sarah began to catch up with her peers physically.

Psychological: Counseling helped Sarah gain self-esteem and manage her anxieties. She became more confident and socially involved.

Case Study 4: Michael

Background: Michael was a sixteen-year-old teenager living in a suburban neighborhood. He was the youngest of two siblings, both of whom had experienced typical pubertal growth.

Michael was a brilliant musician but struggled with poor self-confidence.

Onset of Puberty: By the age of fifteen, Michael had not displayed any signs of puberty. His endocrinologist diagnosed him with hypogonadotropic hypogonadism, a disorder where the body does not create enough hormones to start puberty.

Challenges:

Physical Development: Michael was substantially shorter and less muscular than his peers, which damaged his self-image.

Emotional Impact: The delay in puberty produced mental discomfort. Michael felt embarrassed and frightened about his lack of progress.

Social Challenges: Michael's delayed puberty led to challenges in social interactions, particularly with his male friends who were more physically developed. Interventions: Michael's doctor prescribed testosterone injections to enhance pubertal growth. He also attended counseling sessions to address his mental and social issues.

Outcomes: Medical: The testosterone therapy successfully triggered pubertal development, allowing Michael to develop secondary sexual traits and catch up in growth.

Emotional and Social: Counseling helped Michael establish self-confidence and improve his social connections. He grew more active in school activities and established stronger friendships.

Analysis and Lessons Learned

The case studies of early and late puberty provide useful insights into the issues and solutions associated with unusual pubertal timing. The following analysis emphasizes the major lessons learned.

1. Importance of Early Diagnosis and Intervention Early diagnosis and proper intervention are critical for controlling both early and late puberty. In the cases of Emily and John, early detection of premature puberty allowed for appropriate medical and psychological therapy. Similarly, early detection of delayed puberty in Sarah and Michael provided prompt hormone therapy and psychological assistance.

Lesson: Healthcare practitioners should be cautious in monitoring public growth and swiftly address any variations from regular trends.

2. Holistic Approach to Treatment A holistic strategy that integrates medical, psychological, and social therapies is necessary for addressing the numerous issues of atypical puberty. In all four case studies, the combination of hormone therapy and psychotherapy offered comprehensive assistance.

Lesson: Interventions should address not just the physical components of puberty but also the psychological and social dimensions to guarantee general well-being.

3. Role of Family and School Support

Family and school contexts have a significant role in assisting teenagers through atypical puberty. Emily and John benefited from supportive families and school programs that addressed bullying and encouraged a good atmosphere. Sarah and Michael both got encouragement and understanding from their families and schools. -

Lesson: Families and schools should work together to provide supportive environments that foster good development and address the special requirements of adolescents with abnormal pubertal timing.

4. Addressing Psychological Impact The psychological impact of early or late puberty can be considerable, impacting self-esteem, anxiety levels, and social interactions. Counseling and

psychological support were crucial in helping the individuals in the case studies cope with their emotions and develop resilience.

Lesson: Psychological support should be an integral aspect of the intervention plan for adolescents undergoing atypical puberty.

5. Individualized Treatment Plans Each adolescent's experience with puberty is distinct, demanding specific treatment regimens. The case studies illustrate that individualized therapies, adapted to the specific requirements and circumstances of each individual, are most effective.

Lesson: Healthcare providers should establish tailored treatment regimens that include the physical, emotional, and social context of each adolescent.

The case studies of early and late puberty underline the significance of comprehensive, tailored interventions that address the physical, psychological, and social elements of pubertal development. Early diagnosis and timely intervention, a comprehensive approach to treatment, the importance of family and school support, addressing the psychological impact, and devising tailored treatment plans are all essential aspects of achieving excellent results for adolescents undergoing atypical puberty. By learning from these case studies, healthcare providers, families, and schools can better support adolescents through the challenges of early or late puberty, promoting healthier and more resilient individuals.

Chapter 8.

Public Health Implications

Puberty is a major developmental stage that represents the transition from childhood to adulthood. Puberty is a common developmental stage. As a result of hormonal alterations, this time period is characterized by a number of changes that occur on a physiological, psychological, and emotional level. To ensure the health and happiness of teenagers, it is essential to get an understanding of the public health consequences of puberty and to take steps to address these issues. The importance of screening and early detection of puberty-related issues is discussed in this chapter. Additionally, policy recommendations to support healthy development are outlined, and community and educational programs that are designed to educate and support young people and their families during this crucial stage are discussed.

Screening and Early Detection

• The Importance of Detection at an Early Stage
When it comes to reducing potential health
problems and ensuring that adolescents receive
the right assistance and care, early recognition of
issues associated with puberty is one of the most
important factors. The identification of early or
delayed puberty can assist in the treatment of
underlying health difficulties, the provision of
essential therapies, and the promotion of the
mental and emotional well-being of adolescents.

Screening Method

The various techniques of screening Several
procedures are used to test for puberty-related
disorders, including physical examinations,
growth monitoring, hormone assessments, and
psychological evaluations.

1. Physical Examinations: Regular physical
exams by healthcare practitioners can assess
growth patterns and uncover indicators of early
or delayed puberty. These exams often entail

examining height, weight, and the development of secondary sexual traits.

2. Growth Monitoring: Tracking growth throughout time using growth charts can help spot variations from regular development trends, which may suggest early or delayed puberty.

3. Hormonal Assessments: Blood tests to evaluate hormone levels, such as testosterone, estrogen, and thyroid hormones, can help diagnose puberty-related illnesses. Elevated or inadequate hormone levels can signify issues that need to be addressed.

4. Bone Age Assessment: X-rays of the hand and wrist can measure bone age, offering insights into whether skeletal growth coincides with chronological age. This can assist in identifying early or delayed puberty.

5. Psychological Evaluations: Assessing the mental and emotional well-being of adolescents is vital, as puberty can severely impair psychological health. Screenings for anxiety,

depression, and other mental health concerns help provide prompt support and intervention.

Common Puberty-Related Issues

Several puberty-related issues may necessitate screening and early detection:

1. Precocious Puberty: The early onset of puberty, often before age 8 in girls and age 9 in boys, can lead to emotional and social obstacles and may suggest underlying health issues.

 2. Delayed Puberty: Puberty is termed delayed if there are no symptoms of development by age 13 in girls and age 14 in boys. This delay might be caused by several circumstances, including hormone abnormalities and chronic illnesses.

3. Growth Disorders: Conditions such as growth hormone insufficiency and Turner syndrome can impact growth and development throughout puberty.

4. Menstrual Disorders: Irregular, painful, or heavy menstrual periods might suggest

underlying health concerns and harm an adolescent's quality of life. 5. Mental health disorders: puberty may be a trying time emotionally, and disorders such as anxiety, despair, and body image worries are frequent.

Challenges in Screening

Several obstacles can prevent successful screening for puberty-related issues:

1. Access to Healthcare: Limited access to healthcare services, particularly in low-income and rural areas, might limit early detection and intervention.

2. Stigma and Privacy Concerns: Adolescents may be reluctant to seek help or address puberty-related issues owing to shame or concerns about privacy.

3. Lack of Awareness: Parents and teenagers may not identify the indicators of

puberty-related disorders, delaying the identification and treatment of these issues.

4. Resource Constraints: Healthcare practitioners may confront limits in resources, including time and access to specialist testing, impacting the thoroughness of screenings.

Policy Recommendations

Enhancing access to screening services To address access challenges and ensure early detection of puberty-related problems, the following policy measures should be considered:

1.Invest in Healthcare Infrastructure : Expand healthcare facilities and services, particularly in underserved areas, to offer comprehensive screening and care for adolescents.

2. Train Healthcare Professionals: Implement training programs for healthcare practitioners to ensure they are competent to recognize and handle puberty-related concerns efficiently.

3. Telehealth Services: Utilize telehealth to enhance access to healthcare services, allowing teenagers in distant places to get screenings and consultations without geographical barriers.

4. Subsidize Screening Costs : Provide financial support or subsidies to make screening services affordable for all families, particularly those with little financial resources.

Promoting public awareness and education

Public awareness and education are crucial for encouraging early detection and adequate care of puberty-related issues.

1. Public Awareness Campaigns: Launch campaigns to educate parents and adolescents about the indicators of early and delayed puberty, the significance of regular screenings, and accessible resources.

2. School Programs: Integrate health education into school curricula to inform students about

puberty, its stages, and the significance of seeking care for any difficulties.

3. Community Outreach: Engage community groups and leaders to disseminate information and encourage participation in screening programs.

Ensuring Continuity of Care Screening programs must be part of a holistic approach to adolescent health.

1. Integrated Health Systems: Develop integrated health systems that ensure seamless transitions from screening to diagnosis, treatment, and follow-up care.

2. Electronic Health Records : Implement electronic health records to maintain adolescents' health data, improve continuity of care, and track progress.

3. Patient Navigation Services: Provide patient navigation services to help adolescents and their families comprehend screening results and

navigate the healthcare system for subsequent care.

Addressing stigma and privacy concerns

Reducing stigma and preserving privacy can encourage more adolescents to seek care for puberty-related issues. 1. "Discreet Services": Ensure that healthcare services for adolescents are discreet and respectful of their privacy.

2. Cultural Sensitivity Training: Train healthcare workers to be culturally sensitive and non-judgmental when discussing puberty-related issues with adolescents.

3. Peer Support Programs: Develop peer support programs that allow adolescents to express their experiences and concerns in a safe and supportive atmosphere.

Community and Educational Programs :Role of Community Programs

Community initiatives play a significant role in assisting adolescents through puberty by providing education, resources, and support.

1. Increasing Accessibility: Bring healthcare services and educational activities to communities, particularly those with restricted access to healthcare facilities.

2. Building Trust: Establish trust throughout the community to encourage teenagers and their families to participate in screening programs and seek treatment when needed.

3. Providing Education: Offer education and information regarding puberty, its stages, and the necessity of early detection and intervention for related issues.

4. Supporting Navigation: Assist teenagers and their families in navigating the healthcare system to ensure they obtain appropriate follow-up care and support.

Successful Community Program Models

Several models have been useful in supporting teenagers through puberty:

1. Community Health Workers (CHWs): CHWs are trusted members of the community who give health education, conduct screenings, and aid with follow-up care. Their tight relationships with the community make them useful in encouraging participation in screening programs.

2. School-based Health Programs: Schools can provide a convenient and trusted location for health education and screening services. School nurses and counselors can play a vital role in monitoring students' growth and giving support.

3. Youth Centers and Clubs: Youth centers and clubs can provide a secure location for adolescents to learn about puberty, express their concerns, and seek screening services.

4. Parent Education Programs: Educating parents about puberty and its related challenges can

empower them to support their children during this vital stage.

Educational Programs

Education is a key instrument for promoting public health and assisting teenagers through puberty.

1.   School-based   Programs: Integrate comprehensive health education into school curricula to inform students about puberty, its stages, and the necessity of getting care for any difficulties.

2.   Workshops   and   Seminars: Organize workshops and seminars for parents, teachers, and community members to educate them on puberty-related difficulties and how to support teenagers.

3. Public Awareness Campaigns: Use mass media, social media, and community outreach programs to convey information about puberty and the necessity of early identification and intervention.

4. Healthcare Provider Training: Train healthcare practitioners to effectively communicate with adolescents and their families about puberty-related difficulties, ensuring they feel supported and understood.

Measuring impact and outcomes To ensure the effectiveness of community and educational programs, it is vital to monitor their impact and outcomes.

1. Data Collection: Collect data on participation rates, screening outcomes, and follow-up care to evaluate the success of programs.

2. Surveys and Feedback: Use surveys and feedback from participants to examine their knowledge, attitudes, and behaviors addressing puberty-related issues.

3. Long-term Tracking: Track the long-term health outcomes of adolescents who participate in screening programs to establish their impact on general health and well-being.

4. Cost-Benefit Analysis: Conduct cost-benefit assessments to determine the economic impact of screening programs and justify sustained funding and support.

Puberty is a key period of development that can greatly affect an individual's health and well-being. Effective screening and early detection of puberty-related disorders are critical for ensuring that adolescents receive the required assistance and care. Policy proposals should focus on expanding access to screening services, boosting public awareness and education, guaranteeing continuity of care, and addressing stigma and privacy issues. Community and educational programs play a critical role in assisting adolescents through puberty by providing education, resources, and support. By employing these techniques, we can support healthy development and increase the quality of life for teenagers as they traverse this vital stage of life.

Conclusion

Social and developmental Context

The timing of puberty does not occur in isolation; it is impacted by and effects the broader social and developmental milieu. Understanding this setting is critical for thoroughly addressing the implications of early and late puberty. Early Puberty For early-maturing teenagers, the physical changes associated with puberty can lead to complex social interactions. Early-maturing females may receive more attention from boys and adults, which can be overpowering and lead to feelings of vulnerability and anxiety. They may also feel compelled to engage in romantic and sexual relationships before they are emotionally ready. This can result in increased levels of stress and anxiety, hurting their mental health and social interactions. Early-maturing boys may experience social advantages, such as higher popularity and athletic success, but they also face demands to conform to masculine standards. These pressures might lead to dangerous behaviors and mental health difficulties if individuals feel unable to match society's expectations. The social and developmental environment of early puberty demands sophisticated knowledge and specific interventions to support healthy growth. Parental and cultural expectations can also influence the experiences of early-maturing teenagers. Parents may not be prepared to confront the issues of early puberty, resulting in a lack of support and direction. Societal expectations around body appearance and conduct might further complicate the experiences of early-maturing adolescents. Comprehensive education and support systems are important to help parents and teenagers negotiate these issues. Late Puberty For late-maturing adolescents, the delay in physical development can contribute to feelings of alienation and social isolation. Boys who mature late may suffer from feelings of inadequacy and self-consciousness about their lack of muscle development and height, while girls may be apprehensive about their delayed breast development and menstruation. These feelings might damage their self-esteem and mental health, leading to despair and anxiety. Social isolation is a common experience for late-maturing adolescents. The delay in physical development might make it difficult for children to blend in with their peers, resulting in loneliness and a sense of not belonging. This social isolation can contribute to feelings of depression and anxiety, hurting their general well-being. The psychological stress of delayed puberty can also influence academic achievement. Adolescents who are focused on their physical development and social acceptance may find it difficult to concentrate on their education. Stress and anxiety might undermine their motivation and involvement in school, potentially hurting their academic accomplishments. Concerns about future reproductive health can weigh heavily on late-maturing teens. The ambiguity regarding their sexual development and potential fertility concerns can cause great distress. Addressing these concerns through medical intervention and psychological assistance is vital for their mental well-being. Conclusion The time of puberty, whether early or late, has important ramifications for both mental and physical health. Early puberty is associated with an increased risk of obesity, cardiovascular diseases, bone health issues, and mental health disorders, while late puberty is linked to delayed growth and development, decreased bone density, reproductive health concerns, and psychological stress. The social and developmental environment of puberty further complicates these experiences, altering the mental and physical health outcomes of teenagers.To encourage healthy development, it is vital to raise knowledge about the implications of early and late puberty and execute focused treatments. Comprehensive education and support systems are important to help parents, healthcare providers, and adolescents negotiate the obstacles of puberty. By addressing the physical and mental health consequences of

pubertal timing, we can improve the well-being of adolescents and ensure they receive the support and care they need during this key phase of development.

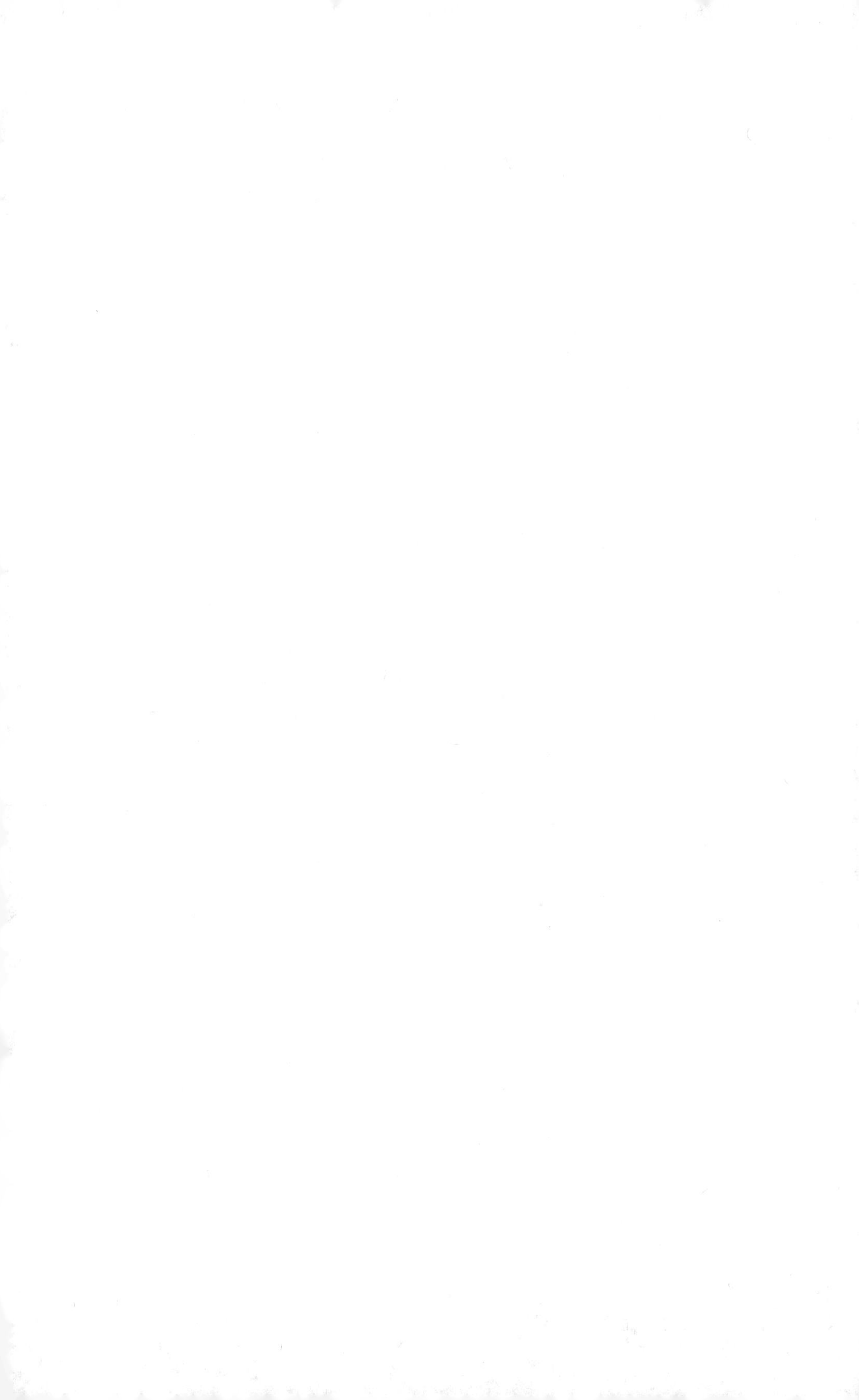

www.ingramcontent.com/pod-product-compliance
Lightning Source LLC
Chambersburg PA
CBHW071037250726

48653CB00005B/1867